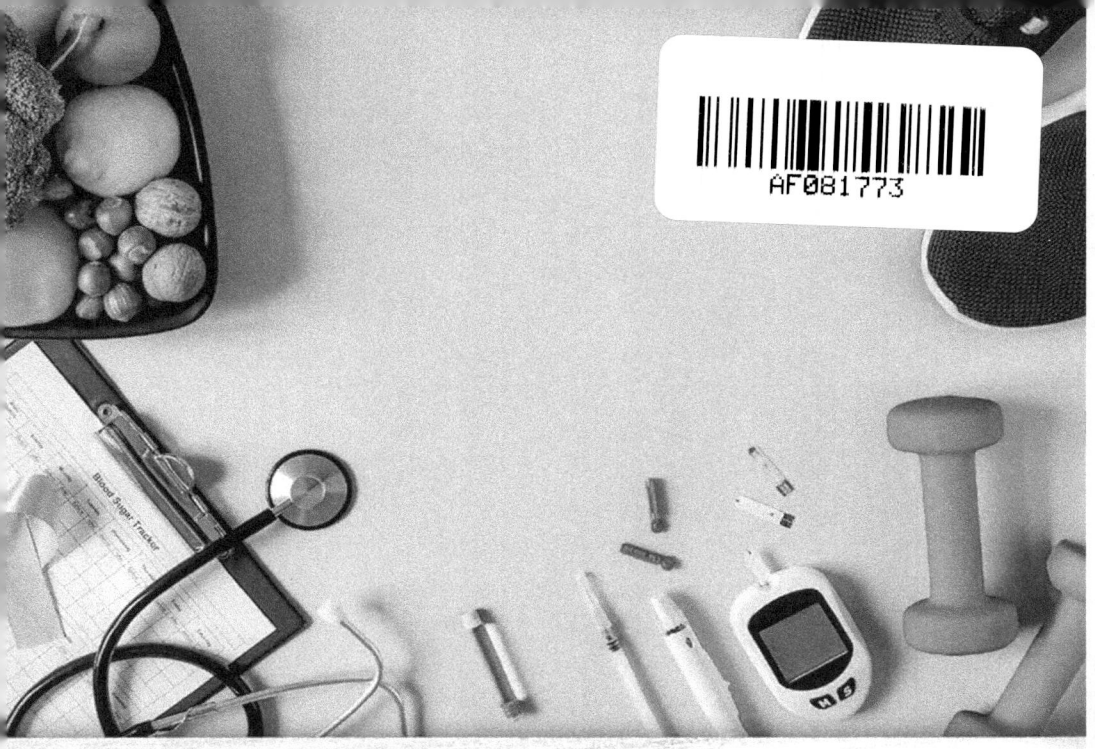

BEATING
Diabetes
TODAY

YOUR ROAD MAP TO CONTROL, SAVINGS, AND RECOVERY

LAMAR PHILLIPS

Copyright © 2024 by Lamar Phillips

ISBN: 978-1-77883-357-1 (Paperback)

978-1-77883-358-8 (Hardback)

978-1-77883-359-5 (E-book)

All rights reserved. No part of this publication may be reproduced, distributed, or transmitted in any form or by any means, including photocopying, recording, or other electronic or mechanical methods, without the prior written permission of the publisher, except in the case brief quotations embodied in critical reviews and other noncommercial uses permitted by copyright law.

The views expressed in this book are solely those of the author and do not necessarily reflect the views of the publisher, and the publisher hereby disclaims any responsibility for them. Some names and identifying details in this book have been changed to protect the privacy of individuals.

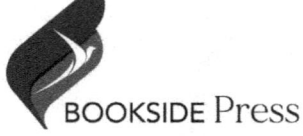

BookSide Press
877-741-8091
www.booksidepress.com
orders@booksidepress.com

Contents

My Story vii
    Greetings Dear Reader vii
    My Song ix
    Unnecessary Tragedy x
I. Understanding Diabetes xiii
    Important Information For Diabetics xiv
Section One: Background And Medical Statistics Of Type 2 Diabetes 1
    Important Statistics Regarding the Prevalence of Diabetes in the Human Race 1
Section Two: Causes Of Type 2 Diabetes 5
    Description of Types 1 and 2 Diabetes 5
    Symptoms of Type 2 Diabetes 7
    Contributors to Type 2 Diabetes 8
    Diseases Caused by Type 2 Diabetes 9
Section Three: How To Reduce Blood Sugar Count, Reverse The Disease, And Apply The Principal Medications 13
Section Four: Methods And Techniques For Improving The Use Of Diabetic Instruments And Lowering Their Costs ... 17
    Pricking Methods 17
    Pricking Techniques 19
    Handling of Test Strips 21
    Insulin Injection Methods 22
    Insulin Injection Techniques 24
    Use of Needles 24
    Conclusion 27

II. Whipping Diabetes..29
- The Danger of Overdosing.....................................29
- Relating to Non-Diabetic Meals...............................32
- How You Get Diabetes..34
- How to Get Rid of Diabetes....................................41
- The 10 best diabetes-friendly foods 45
- The Truth about the Proper Cure for Diabetes 47
- How to Get Rid of Neuropathy Pain............................48
- How to Live Longer 50

My Story, Continued..55
- Remembering..55

My Song, Final..59
MY SONG by Lamar Phillips 61

Discover how to keep your diabetes under control, how to save tons of money, and best of all, how to get rid of it.

Lamar Phillips tells his story of how he took all three of these important steps. It's a story that'll highly inspire you to do the same.

It's one of the greatest booklets on diabetes recovery ever to be written.

HOW TO REDUCE DIABETES COSTS
(And how to reverse it ----- the disease)

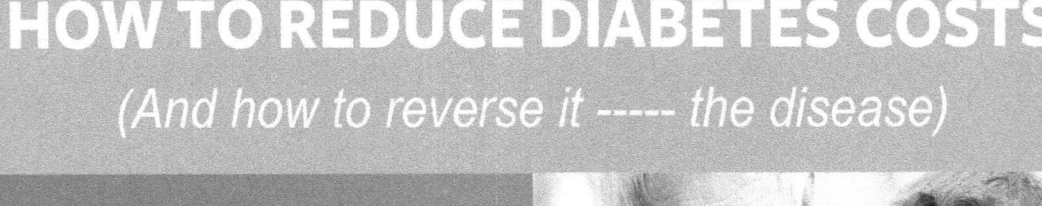

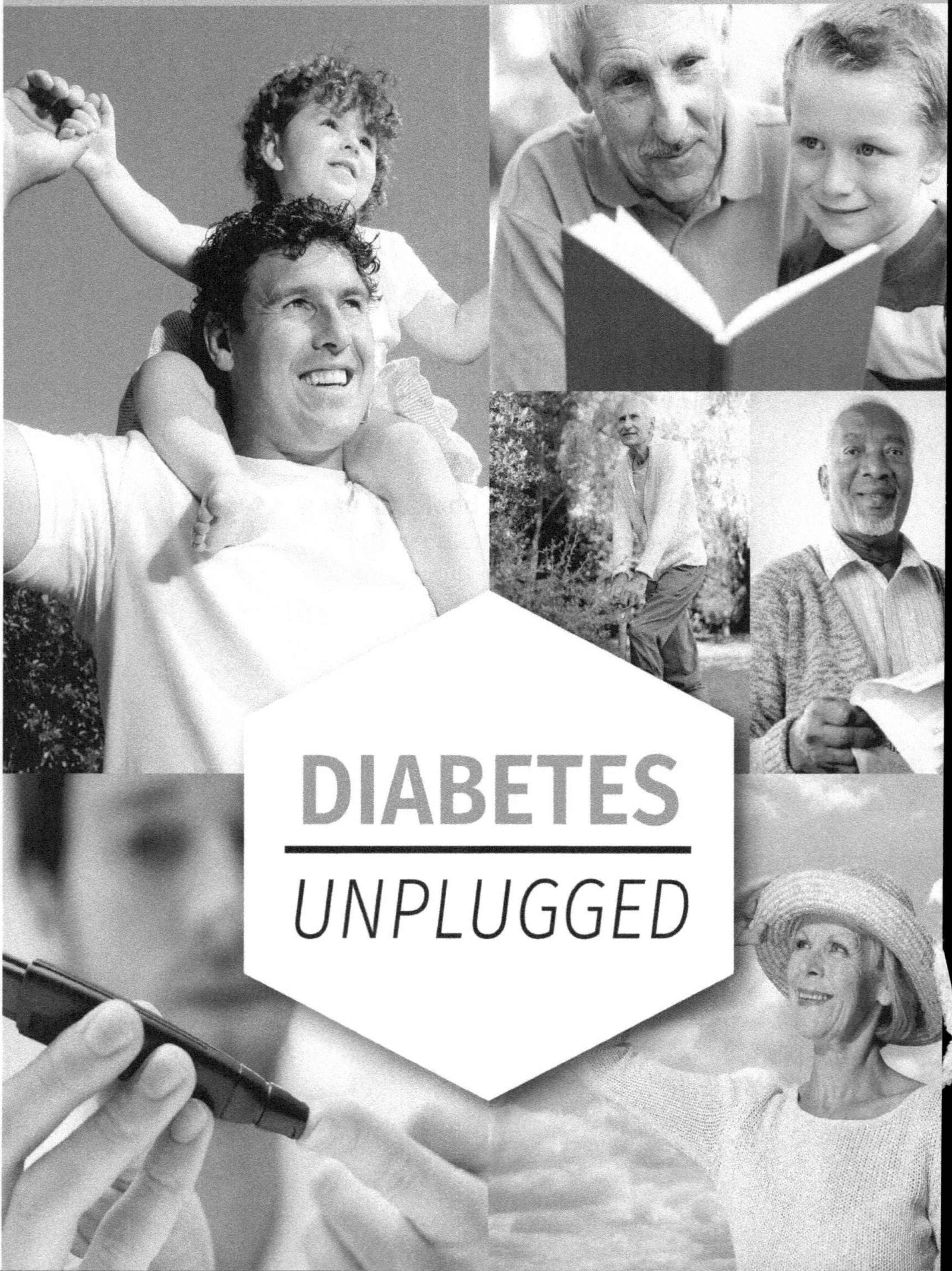

DIABETES
UNPLUGGED

MY STORY

P**lease be aware:** In targeting Type 2 diabetics, which include children, youth, middle age, and seniors, it has became clear that a sophisticated style of writing and the use of technical terms would limit this book to only the highly educated and avid-reader class who are readily familiar with such language, and therefore eliminate a large segment of diabetics, especially the youth and others who have a different lifestyle and are not prone to read lengthy treatises, even when it has to do with their disease.

Of course, I don't contemplate children 8 to 12 reading and studying this book on their own, since they will be instructed and monitored mainly by their parents. But a short, easy-to-read book will make it much easier for all classes to understand the complications of Type 2 and what they need to do to keep it under control and how to manage lancets and needles. Thus, I'm writing this book in a style that is easy and clear reading for almost everybody with diabetes.

Greetings Dear Reader

As the author of this article and as a former diabetic, I am pleased to share my story—about how I got it, how I deal with it, and how I saved money. Now, I want to tell you how my experience can help you better understand it and successfully combat it. I can clearly remember how, during my young, middle age, and later years, the one thing I dreaded and prayed that I would never get, was diabetes. You see, my brother's wife had diabetes. She came down with it when she was 27 years old. She began feeling tired all the time and was having difficulty seeing properly. When she was diagnosed with type 1 diabetes, a disease that can't be cured, she immediately put into action the standard strategies for controlling diabetes that doctors recommended. She actually lived till she was 63, a miracle, her doctor said, because normally those with type 1 never made it to that age at that time. But she survived many years longer than most type 1's do because she was highly disciplined. But her case only made me more afraid than ever of possibly contracting it myself.

However, during her life the only types of needles available were the very long ones. It was before the development of Flexpens and Kwikpens. When I watched my sister in law self-inject with those long pens in various parts of her body, and the pain she went through, I was aghast. You see, it wasn't only the pain, but the regime of daily injections, regulating the diet, and the potential for the various diseases that occur from diabetes that frightened me. I prayed I would never get it. But I had one defect: I loved sweet things. Now, don't get me wrong. I wasn't a sodaholic or a cookieholic like countless prediabetics are who drink many soft drinks every day, both at meals and in-between them, and are heavy on pastas, potatoes, and butter and oils, chocolates, and various types of cookies. No, I wasn't heavy on any of these things. In fact, I seldom drank sodas and was fair on the other items.

So I can hear you saying, "how, then, did you get it?" Good question. First of all, since I was about 27, I was overweight, not a lot, but about 25 pounds. Then when I got into my forties, I went up from around 175 to nearly 200, and I stayed that way for years and years, till I was 71; and at that time I was 60 pounds more than the weight I should have had for my height. On top of my overweight problem, I loved to have something sweet with my meals, not a lot, but just one cookie or maybe also a few raisins or the like, per meal, especially when I was away from home for the day, which I frequently was. On top of this, I loved white potatoes and frequent spaghettis and various macaronis, but again, not humungous servings. At that time my wife and I were living overseas in Albania. In that country the almost exclusive bread available was made of white flour and since it contained sourdough, I loved it and ate some every day.

As you can see, it wasn't anything massive I was doing. I wasn't grossly overweight (60 pounds—many diabetics are 100 pounds or more overweight) or a humongous ingester of carbohydrates and sweet drinks.

My big problem was the long-term consistency of first being overweight, and second, consistently—day after day, year after year—eating sweet things in small portions. And there was a third element—not enough exercise. My work was mainly administrative. I did, however, work in the garden around our house, a hobby I loved, but it wasn't very strenuous.

Of course, it was bound to happen, but I had no inkling of such a result. It didn't even occur to me. Diabetes was only for those gross abusers. But then I started feeling tired upon rising in the mornings, and I continued with that feeling all day long. After a few months, I went to a local doctor. He took my blood sugar count and found it was around 140, which was more than two hours after my lunch that day.

His diagnosis? Prediabetes. He counseled me to be careful with my diet. But since he didn't speak loud and clear of where I was headed if I didn't make substantial changes, I didn't take him seriously.

My Song

One year later, in the fall of 2009, we took our vacation to the United States, our native country. As we usually did on our vacations, we visited our family doctor. I was very intent on getting her diagnosis of my unrelenting tiredness and the uncomfortable feelings that were developing in my feet.

Well, you guessed it! She immediately took my blood sugar count, and I was blown away! It was 350! No wonder I had been feeling so tired all the time. She checked my feet. Neuropathy was setting in! Boy was I scared. She immediately put me to bed in her clinic, and I stayed there for several days till she and the nurses were able to get the count down to a normal level.

What I remember worst about that experience was the day the nurse came into my room with a needle in her hand. I said, "What's that for?" She answered, "For your diabetes." "No," I yelled. "That's not for me. I don't need that. Go away." "Yes you do. This is what the doctor has ordered," she said.

I wanted to get out of that bed and run. Me? Taking injections everyday for the rest of my life? No way! But what could I do? In my condition it was impossible to run. You see. It hit me right there—the thing I had dreaded all my life had actually happened, and there was nothing I could do about it, at least not at that moment! I can't describe the horrible feeling I had that day.

Later, the doctor told me that I would live longer if I took the injection and not the pill—the Metformin. Why? Because each time one measures one's blood sugar count, one can adjust the dosage to fit the count; and that can't be done so easily with a pill.

So where am I now with my diabetes? That's another story that I'll share with you later on. But I will tell you one thing—it's now nine years later, and I'm 80 at this writing and going strong, got all my marbles, work several hours in my yard and garden every day, write articles for magazines, and actually look at least ten years younger than I really am!

Unnecessary Tragedy

Back in 2013 I became acquainted with a young man who was perhaps 22 or 23 years old. He drove a very nice pickup truck and did some small jobs for me. He looked healthy and didn't seem to be limited in what he could do physically. I was impressed. It turned out that he lived with his parents next door to one of my sons. Some two months passed after he did the last job for me. Then one day when my son was visiting me, I asked him how that young man was doing.

"Oh," he said, "didn't you know he died?"

What? Is it true?" I exclaimed. I was stunned. "What happened?"

"His parents found him dead behind their house one night. He had gone outside to do an errand, and he never came back. Upon checking, they found him lying on the ground, gone."

What I learned was that he was diabetic and had been totally ignoring the health rules required for controlling the disease. He drank many, many sodas every day, ate carbohydrates like crazy, and oily and fatty foods without restraint, and in short, took no controlling measures whatsoever. As a result, his heart quit beating. A sad case? Absolutely. But you see, it can happen sooner or later to anyone, maybe even to you, if you live that kind of a life style. Yes, it may not be so drastic, such as loss of vision, a destroyed kidney, or neuropathy so bad you can't walk anymore, when you totally ignore the eating behavior needed to keep it under control.

UNDERSTANDING DIABETES

Diabetes types 1 and 2 are serious diseases, which can lead to dreadful symptoms; and, if not carefully controlled, can ultimately cause death. Additionally, for those using lancets, test strips, and pen needles for insulin injections, the cost can be very high, not only for those rendering a co-pay with Medicare and/or other insurance coverages, but even worse for those with little or no insurance coverage. In this testament, you will learn how to:

- Better control your diabetes;
- Reduce costs;
- Improve the use of injection needles, lancets and test strips;
- How to Reverse Diabetes Type 2.

This testimony by me, a sufferer of diabetes, and others, is divided into four sections.

- Section 1 gives a brief background and medical statistics of type 2 diabetes.
- Section 2 explains the causes, description, and nature of types 1 & 2.
- Section 3 explains how to reduce your blood sugar count, and how you can control and/or reverse type 2 diabetes.

- Section 4 explains how to improve use of the injection needles, lancets and test strips.

Important Information For Diabetics

If you have type 1 or type 2 diabetes, this information can drastically reduce your medical costs and also better control your disease. Medical reduction costs are based on reliable testimonies that are indirectly included here.

As most diabetics know, the cost of injection needles, lancets, and test strips are extremely expensive. **This is just one of the main purposes for sharing this information with you.** But first, there is other important related information about types 1 and 2 diabetes that you should read. For the moderately fast reader, these sixty-one pages can be read in approximately 30 to 45 minutes. All sections are supremely important, as they can significantly improve your health, if seriously applied, and drastically reduce costs.

SECTION ONE

Background And Medical Statistics Of Type 2 Diabetes

I suggest you read all this material carefully, because acquiring a clear understanding is key to applying correctly what is recommended here and for understanding how to reduce costs.

Note: Unfortunately, type 1 diabetes is an irreversible disease and cannot be cured, but type 2 can be cured, often referred to as reversed. And the cost of types 1 and 2 medical instruments can be drastically reduced. Methods for reducing these costs are discussed in *Section 4*.

Important Statistics Regarding the Prevalence of Diabetes in the Human Race

Statistics for diabetes in the world for 2021

- There were 537 million people ages 20—79 in the world with diabetes in 2021.
- 1 in 10 adults in the world had diabetes in 2021.
- Three quarters of people with diabetes live in low and middle income countries.

Lamar Phillips

Statistics for Diabetes in the United States for 2021.

- 26.9 million new cases were diagnosed.
- 210,000 children and adolescents younger than age 20 years—or 25 per 10,000 youths—had diabetes. This includes 187,000 with type 1 diabetes.
- 1.4 million adults aged 20 years or older reported having type 1 diabetes and using insulin.
- About 208,000 Americans under age 20 (youth) were estimated to have diabetes, approximately 25% of that population number.
- Diabetes kills more Americans than HIV/AIDS and breast cancer combined.

Statistics according to race in the United States in 2021.

- American Indians and Alaskan natives were the highest with diabetes—14.7%.
- Hispanics followed with 12.5%
- Blacks were next at 11%.
- Asians were at 9.2%.
- Whites were at 7.5%.

Statistics according to age and death in 2021.

- 96 million adults, ages 18 or older, living in the United States had pre-diabetes in 2019 (latest statistic).
- 34.2 million persons of all ages living in the United States had diabetes in 2020 according to Center for Disease Control.
- 37.4% of those with diabetes in 2020 were men.
- 29.2% of those with diabetes in 2020 were women.
- 416,000 persons in the United States died of diabetes

in 2021.
- Of all countries in the world, China has the highest diabetes rates.
- The international cost of diabetes in 2021 was $966 billion. This is about 15% of the global cost of health.
- 215.2 million men in the world had diabetes.
- 199.5 million women in the world had diabetes.
- 1.4 million new cases of Americans are diagnosed with diabetes every year.
- Every 6 seconds someone dies from diabetes.
- 642 million people in the world are expected to have the disease in 2040.

NOTE: Some of the above statics may vary according to the Internet source.

SECTION TWO

CAUSES OF TYPE 2 DIABETES

- *Too much oil and grease in the diet.* Most Americans are eating too much fried foods, such as meat, French fries, hamburgers, butter, mayonnaise, peanut butter, etc., which add too much fat to the diet.
- *Too much sugar in the diet.* The majority of Americans are also drinking and eating very sugary soft drinks and too sweet fruit juices, as well as desserts, canned foods with added sugar, refined carbohydrates (white bread, crackers, white rice; and pastas, such as spaghetti, macaroni, etc., and potatoes), which add weight to the body.
- *Too little exercise.* Because of the urban life style, millions of Americans are not getting enough physical exercise. Sufficient exercise burns excess fat, but when the excess fat is not burned, unnecessary weight is added to the body, contributing to diabetes.

Description of Types 1 and 2 Diabetes

In a nutshell, type 2 diabetes can be described in the following way: The human body is composed of cells, the majority of which are located on the exterior of the body. The cells make up muscles and other tissue. When one eats healthy foods, such as greens and other natural vegetables and modest amounts of oil, grease/fats, carbohydrates, and sugar, the nutrients produced from them are absorbed into the walls of the stomach from the digestive process, and from there the nutrients enter into the blood stream, which carries them to the body cells, primarily to the arms, legs, neck, face, chest, back and stomach. A primary component of the dietary system is insulin, a hormone produced by beta cells in the pancreas that regulates the movement of glucose (sugar) into the cells. It is this hormone—insulin—that opens the cells, thus allowing the nutrients that come from the stomach into the blood to enter and properly feed and maintain the body tissue.

However, and this is very important to understand, when too much fat from oily and sugary foods is consumed, the cells start clogging from the fat, preventing the insulin from opening and allowing the nutrients to enter. Since the cells can't absorb the nutrients, the blood, that can't dispose of the glucose and other nutrients, becomes over laden with the glucose (produced by the liver), and two immediate results follow:

1) The body, for a lack of nutrients, tires easily; and 2) the blood, because of too high content of glucose, causes various diseases in the body. The solution is a change of diet, with less of these unhealthful foods. How does one know if diabetes is starting to develop in the body? The principal way to discover the approaching disease is to measure the blood sugar count both in the morning before breakfast, and again two hours after breakfast. The same should be done for each meal, and again before bedtime, for at least three days. Your doctor can do these tests for you or provide the medical instruments for their application. The average healthy blood sugar count (BSC) is 90—110. Usually the BSC rises to 140—160 after meals in a normally healthy person, when modest amounts of sugary drinks and servings of carbohydrates have been consumed. In a healthy person, the BSC drops rapidly back to normal after two hours.

However, when the BSC is still high after two hours—say 150—160 or higher—this then indicates there is diabetes in the works.

Furthermore, when diabetes is developing as a result of long-time consummation of sugary drinks, carbohydrates, and oily foods, and one is overweight, the count can rise higher than 160—it can even shoot up to 350 and sometimes to 600 or above, which is extremely dangerous—and remain there for several hours; and if in the morning and at bedtime, the count is considerably above 110 (when it should be under 100), and you are running consistently 150 or above, you are either with pre-diabetes or with full-time diabetes. If this is the case, you should see a doctor immediately.

So, remember, in type 2 diabetes, the pancreas continues to produce insulin, but the insulin can't penetrate the body cells because they are blocked. In type 1 diabetes, the pancreas discontinues producing insulin at different ages of the person, some at a very young age and others at a later date, but seldom does it stop producing in older persons.

How does one know if diabetes is starting to develop in the body? You will probably first start feeling tired consistently, even after a good night's sleep, then even during the day and into the evening. You may also begin to feel numbness in the front of the bottom of your feet. Below are the various symptoms of type 2 diabetes.

Symptoms of Type 2 Diabetes

Diabetes symptoms will vary from person to person, and not all the symptoms listed below will likely affect a person. The important indication to watch for is continuation of the symptom(s). If you feel anyone of them or several on an on-going basis, then you need to consult your physician immediately.

- Extreme thirst.
- Frequent urination.
- Drowsiness or lethargy.
- Increased appetite.

- Sudden weight loss.
- Sudden vision changes.
- Sugar in the urine (discovered through blood tests).
- Fruity, sweet or wine-like odor on the breath.
- Heavy or labored breathing.
- Stupor or unconsciousness (caused by extremely low or high blood count).
- Numbness in the toes.

Contributors to Type 2 Diabetes

Up until the 1980s and 1990s, type 2 diabetes was not a serious medical concern. In fact, few Americans had type 2 diabetes. What, then, caused the dramatic increases in the disease? There are at least four reasons.

- ***The change from farm to city.*** Until the 1900s, the majority of Americans were rural dwellers. In fact, in 1900, 50% of Americans were living outside the cities. By 2000, only 1% were living in the countryside. As farmers and country citizens, there was considerably more physical activity and a broader vegetable diet, since much of the food was produced in family gardens and from commercial crops, both of which required lots of physical labor and a good supply of non-fat and low-in-sugar foods. Natural foods and physical exercise are known to be major deterrents to diabetes.
- ***The change from natural foods to processed foods.*** Beginning as far back as the 1960s, the food industry began modifying their products to include, whenever possible, glucose (sugar) in their products. Now, in the 2000s, almost all canned and prepared foods contain

sugar, some more, some less. The purpose, of course, is to increase sales since the human being normally likes a sweet taste. Sugar, in excessive amounts, is one of the primary causes of diabetes. Before the 1960s, most people ate mostly non-processed foods. Now probably 80% of people's diet is processed foods.

- *The rise of fast food restaurants.* Beginning in the 1960s, the number of restaurants serving delicious, but non-healthy, food began to rise dramatically. Centered first in the larger cities of the nation, today they can be found in even the smallest towns and villages across the country in many nations of the world. Because of their high savory, they have become a melting pot for people of all ages, especially for youth and young adults, who usually continue such a debilitating diet into their middle and senior years. Sugary drinks, white foods, refined carbohydrates (bread, crackers, pastas, etc.) and those that contain high levels of oil and grease, which convert to fat, seriously contribute to diabetes.
- *The decline of the middle class.* Since the middle 1970s and early 1980s, the middle class in America has been declining, due to the refusal of the American industry to continue raising wages and salaries appropriately to the American worker. With inadequate income, most American families in this category have had to subsist on a substandard, less expensive diet, a diet filled with sugar and fat.

Diseases Caused by Type 2 Diabetes

Diabetes, if not controlled, can eventually cause five major health problems.

- ***Blindness.*** This frightful problem will not occur at once, but will slowly dim the eyes over a period of several years, and the more serious the disease, the sooner will blindness (technically called glaucoma) occur. It can even happen in an instant when the disease is far along, perhaps while driving, while hiking, while eating, or sleeping, or studying. It can happen under any circumstances.
- ***Heart Failure.*** Diabetes can weaken the heart and eventually cause an attack that the subject may perchance survive, but with permanent damage; or it can cause instant death, or provoke cardiac arrest, a phenomenon in which the heart simply stops beating, sometimes, however, with no pain.
- ***Kidney Failure.*** One kidney can fail before the other, or both can simultaneously deteriorate until a transplant is necessary. The disturbing fact, regarding this situation, is that the demand for kidneys is so high that the waiting list is enormous; thus, receiving one for a transplant is very remote for many people. The other solution is to take dialysis, which usually is required up to three times a week for six hours each treatment, which for most persons, especially those living in remote areas, is a major challenge; and if one is not covered by insurance, the cost can be prohibitive.
- ***Neuropathy.*** The primary early symptom (along with tiredness) of this problem is manifested in the feet, which begin to lose their feeling. The patient may first feel tingling, then some pain, and finally numbness. Usually the problem occurs first in the bottom front part of the feet, and if not controlled by a proper diet, the numbness will creep into the rest of the feet, and finally up the legs, and sometimes into the hands and arms. Even with a complete

reversal of the disease, *neuropathy is almost impossible to reverse,* but it can be stopped from worsening.
- **Impotence.** According to scientific studies, type 2 diabetes contributes to impotence, meaning men lose their ability to have an erection. This can be traumatic for men and spouses.

SECTION THREE

How To Reduce Blood Sugar Count, Reverse The Disease, And Apply The Principal Medications

Nearly all who are diabetic contracted the disease as a result of dietary abuse—too much sugar, too much fat. Usually the disease came about from long-term practice of eating too much of tasty, but not always good, food; plus drinks and desserts. All diabetics will agree that it is difficult to break these long-time eating habits. In fact, diet is the most difficult life pattern to mend. From my own experience, I know this for a fact. And I know you do, too.

Notwithstanding the difficulty of changing one's diet, it must be done, or anyone of the five symptoms listed above will certainly take place, and some can lead to death. One of the worst offenders which cause high blood sugar count is sweet, sugary drinks taken with a meal or in-between meals. Just eliminating a sugary drink at meal times or in-between will significantly reduce high blood sugar count. Also, eating very small servings of white rice, potatoes, white bread, milk, fruits, and pastas at a meal will add to the drop in BSC.

The best practice is to eat only *one* of these per meal, in a *small serving*. Many Americans are slaves of white bread. Dropping white bread will add to the reduction of BSC. Eliminating dairy butter in exchange for low-fat or no-fat margarines, and selecting cooking oils with low fat content will further reduce the BSC. Ice-cream, cookies, cakes, and other desserts don't need to be entirely eliminated, but should be eaten conservatively, in very small portions, once or twice a week, and not at every meal or between.

Fiber is another dietary ingredient that is important for controlling the disease. A diabetic should eat lots of fiber, such as potato and apple skins, beans, unrefined grains, vegetables, herbs, and the like. Look for dry cereals that advertise high fiber content. Just making these changes will enormously reduce the BSC, bring back new energy, and give a whole new feel to the body.

Exercise is also essential. In today's American culture, aside from athletes and exercise fanatics, most people don't get much exercise at all. It's to work and back, to the table, to the TV, then to bed. Sufficient exercise is another important remedy for lowering the BSC.

In reality, it takes both—a changed diet AND exercise—to reverse type 2 diabetes; but a change of diet is the most important.

Dietary Substitutes. Though it is difficult to make a major change of diet after years of subjection to one type, it can be done, especially since today there are many kosher ways to add flavor to foods that are not readily palatable to the taste. For example:

- **Breads**—substituting white bread for whole wheat or a mix of whole wheat bread with other grains (oats, barley, flax, millet, buckwheat, etc.) will reduce the BSC.
- **Vegetables**—cooked or roasted, such as mushrooms, onions, eggplant, tomatoes, green beans, cooked beans, Brussel sprouts, broccoli, carrots (in small portions, as they have lots of sugar) and zucchini are great for controlling diabetes.
- **Greens**—kale, spinach, chard, collards, mustard greens,

lettuce and cabbage, to name a few—are also very important for bringing a diabetic back to a normal blood count.
- **Drinks**—water is the best, but tea without sugar, though with some lemon and cinnamon stock, will not be counterproductive. Whatever is drunk should be done in small portions, since too much liquid will dilute the digestive juices and prevent those juices from doing their work, which can stop the digestive process and allow the food to ferment, causing indigestion or acid reflux.
- **A moderate serving** of sweet potatoes, which contain fiber, can substitute for white potatoes. Whole wheat pastas, also in moderation, can substitute for white flour pastas, but should be eaten in small portions, all cooked in various and tasty ways, which a clever housewife or spouse can accomplish, and which will surprise even the most difficult new taste learner. In short, all greens and leafy vegetables are strong contributors to the reduction of BSC.

In the end, it is a matter of determination and persistence!

Principal Medications. Most diabetics start out using Metformin, a capsule, as the principal medication, which is orally ingested. However, as the disease progresses for lack of adequate control, in about 10 or more years, the patient will have to switch to liquid insulin injections. Some diabetics may take up to 15 or 20 years, or less, *if they have survived that long*, to switch to the injection procedure. But this transfer can be halted if the patient will take control of the disease by following the instructions listed in this section. Indeed, even the use of Metformin can be terminated by applying these important steps.

SECTION FOUR

Methods And Techniques For Improving The Use Of Diabetic Instruments And Lowering Their Costs

For those diabetics taking insulin by injection, this section will explain the various methods and techniques of a) sourcing blood for measuring one's blood sugar level, b) applying blood on the test strip, c) managing the test strips, and d) injecting insulin into the body. If the diabetic is a small child, and unable to carry out these functions by him or herself, an older, responsible and capable person will obviously have to do it.

Pricking Methods

- ***Method One—Single Site.*** In order to measure the glucose level of the blood, one must draw a sample from someplace in the body. Usually this is done by pricking one of the fingers. Though in the beginning it is somewhat painful, after a number of pricks, for some diabetics, the discomfort usually subsides. But it is important to change fingers from prick to prick in order to avoid the development of calluses.

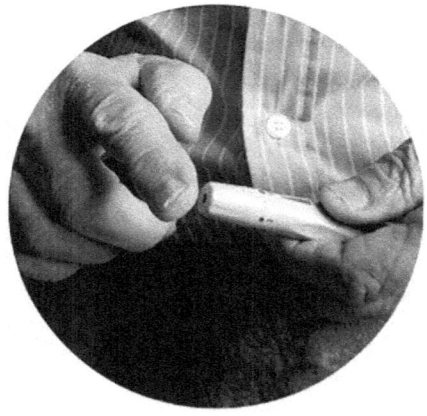

Personally, I have injected into my right hand index fingertip probably at least 5,000 times, and I currently feel no pain whatsoever from an injection in that finger, and there is no hard callous developing. But this may not be the case for many others.

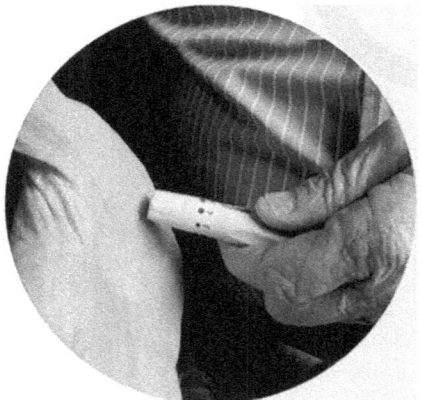

- *Method Two—Multiple Sites.* Aside from the fingers, there are many other places one can prick for blood, such as the tummy and the arms. Some places are less painful than others; though less tender and more easily accessible, they are not always the least painful; but it is good to experiment in order to find the least tender places.

Pricking Techniques

- ***Technique One—Single Use.*** In the diabetic industry, the needle used for pricking is called a lancet. In the medical industry, the lancet is used only one time, primarily to avoid any possible contamination that could result from more than one use. A patient who would become ill or have a sore develop from a contaminated needle could sue the medical personnel or institution involved in the multiple use; and this is the principal reason medical personnel use it only once.

A person who self injects in his or her own private home is not subject to legal action; thus, there is no legal risk in personal multiple injections.

Technique Two—Multiple Use Directly to the Skin. Some diabetics have opted to use the same lancet more than once. In fact, some use it 50 or more times, directly to the skin, without ever experiencing any contamination. I have used it as many as 100 or more times without any negative reactions. Caution should be taken, however, not to prick if the skin is dirty and contaminated with any foreign substance, such as grease, heavy sweat, or any questionable, unclean substance.

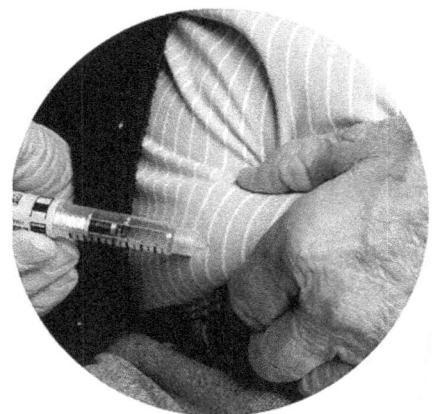

Cleaning or sterilizing the lancet after or before use is the decision of the user. Those I know of who never clean or sterilize after use have never had adverse effects, even after reusing it dozens of times. And personally, after using a lancet dozens of times without cleaning or sterilizing it, I have never had any sores or illness develop from it.

Device Savings. That you may have an idea of costs for medical devices, listed below are samples of original medical devices costs, excluding insurance coverages that have, in my case, been charged to me.

Lancet Pricking Apparatus: $20.00
Lancets per box of 100: $30.00 (30 cents ea.)
Test Strips, each: $1.00
Calibrator Solution, per bottle: $12.00
Kwikpen Injection Pens, each: $27.21
Kwikpen needles, each: $0.52
Note: *Prices may vary among providers.*

As can be quickly calculated, using 1 lancet per week instead of 28, the savings are substantial: 28 X .30 cents = $8.40; and this number multiplied by 4 weeks is a savings of $33.60, or $403.20 per year.

In regards to injection needles, which cost 52 cents each, if you inject a minimum of only four times per day (Lantus and Humalog in the AM and the same again in the PM) you would inject 28 times per week, at a savings of $14.56, or per month $58.24, and for a year $698.88.

Between lancets and needles, the savings per year would be $1,102.08. For those who are injecting more than 4 times per day, the monthly and yearly savings would be far greater.

Those with limited income and no insurance—or even partial insurance—would feel the economical sting very heavily if they changed lancets and needles every time they pricked and injected.

Handling of Test Strips

- ***Method One.*** There are many manufacturers of test strips. Some strips are larger than others, and some take less blood than others to activate the blood glucose meter. The smaller the strip, the more difficult it is to retrieve it from the canister, especially for children and senior citizens, whose hands and fingers are less dexterous. In this case, the larger strips are better. But you will have to decide.

The company you are buying from may have only one size, and in such a case you will have to decide if you want to change supplier. But bear in mind, some insurance companies may not permit a change. Check with your insurance company to find ***out if their policy allows for a change.***

- ***Method Two.*** The advantage of the small test strips is that they take less blood—sometimes just a drop—to activate them. For those who either must stay with the small strips due to insurance policies, or choose the small strips but have difficulty handling them, it is recommended they use a tweezers to remove them from the canister.
- ***Method Three.*** All test strips are very sensitive to dampness of any kind, and if the bottom or especially the top portion of the strip is accidentally touched by a wet or damp finger, it becomes inactive when inserted into the meter. Thus, it is extremely important to handle them with completely dry hands and fingers if a tweezers is not used.

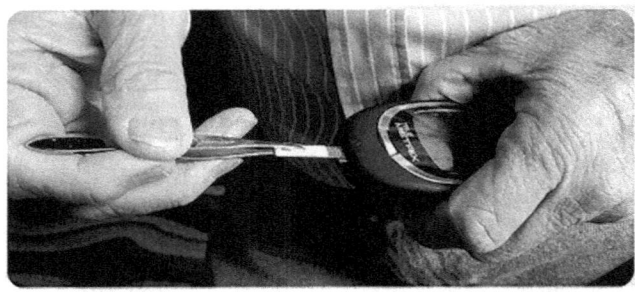

Insulin Injection Methods

- **Method One.** If the sufferer is a small child, and unable to self-inject, an older, responsible and capable person will obviously have to inject. Since today's needles are very short and thin—less than half an inch—the pain is considerably reduced. The stomach, or midsection of the body, is the easiest accessible and the least painful area for injecting. However, there are cases where for some individuals there are other parts of the body which are less tender. It is important to experiment with other areas, if necessary.

Remember that most diabetics of type 2 who begin with Metformin will eventually have to start insulin injections after 10 to 20 years, according to experts in diabetes.

- **Method Two.** If you are a youth, or young or middle-age adult, or a senior citizen, you will be able to self-inject without a problem, providing you are not fearful of injection needles. Some in this category are so fearful of needles that they cannot inject themselves, let alone allow another person to do it. In these cases, it is better for them to take the Metformin tablet, which is orally ingested.

Those of these age groups may wish to experiment, however, with injections to other parts of the body, such as the forearm, the upper leg, or even the buttocks, although this latter area is more difficult to reach.

- ***Method Three.*** Despite the various areas where one may inject oneself, the important factor to remember is that you should not inject yourself in the same spot continually. Doing so will harden that spot—cause a callous—so that it will become impermeable to further injections. It can also become more painful for some persons, since repeated injections can render it more tender; but as I have mentioned above regarding lancets, I and others have not had this problem.

It should be borne in mind that once in a great while the needle will cause a small drop of blood to surface when the needle is withdrawn, and this will make a spot on the clothing. This has happened to me, but rarely. When it does, I use a wet cloth to soak up the blood, and by rubbing it gently with the cloth, the small blood spot disappears, and the wet spot dries in 10 to 15 minutes. I have not let this rare occurrence deter me from injecting through my clothing, since the time saved has been worth it.

Cleaning the injection needle after or before use is the decision of the user. Rarely have those who never clean had adverse effects, even after reusing it dozens of times. I can testify that even with multiple uses without cleaning the needle, I have never had any adverse effects.

Insulin Injection Techniques

- ***Use of Needles—Multiple uses.*** Needles are usually made of high quality metal, meaning they can withstand more than one injection. Some diabetics use the insulin needle 50 times or more. I have used them as many as 150 times.

Some manufacturers of insulin needles claim that just one or two injections will dull the needle so substantially that the point will no longer penetrate easily, and thus cause considerable pain and/or cause a sore that will take time to heal. This may be the case with some needles that may not be of high enough quality to withstand more than one or more injections. You will have to experiment, but for those who repeatedly use a needle of good quality have not experienced undue pain from multiple uses and supposedly dull needles.

Again, however, as in the case of the lancet needles, the insulin injection needle is used only once by medical personnel in order to avoid any risk of contamination and possible legal prosecution by the patient.

Use of Needles

- ***Injection Techniques.*** On the human body, principally in the tummy and where *fat* accumulates mostly, there are three layers: the first one is the epidermis, or outer layer; the second one, the middle layer, is the dermis; and the third one is the hypodermis, where the fat is layered. When one injects in the tummy, depending on how thick the epidermis and dermis are, the needle will usually penetrate only these two outer layers, causing very little pain. However, for those persons who are slender,

with very thin epidermis and dermis layers, if the needle penetrates to the third layer, considerable discomfort will be felt. In order to reduce injection discomfort for those who are very slender, *the needle should be injected at a 90% angle, or more. Squeezing a lump of tummy flesh with one hand and injecting with the other into the lump also helps reduce discomfort.*
- ***Types of Insulin and Their Use.*** As many diabetics know, there are lots of basic types of insulin. Some of the most commonly used ones are:
- Rapid acting—Humalog and Novolog.
- Longer acting (premixed)—Lantus and Levemia.

The purpose of Lantus and Levemia is to help stabilize the blood sugar count, and the purpose of Humalog and Novolog is to quickly reduce an abnormally high sugar count.

These insulin types are marketed in what are called Flexpens or Kwikpens, instruments that contain both the liquid insulin and the needle. The needles of these pens are just slightly over one quarter of an inch long and they can be dialed to the desired dosage, making it very convenient to adjust to the needed amount. After some usage, one can calculate quite effectively the amount of insulin to inject for bringing the count down within one or two hours to the desired level.

Some diabetics inject both types of insulin at the same moment, in order to save time. Personally, I have done it thousands of times. To accomplish this, first remove the cover of the needles, then *hold the two pens between the thumb and forefinger, and simply inject them simultaneously into the desired site.*

Once the needles are injected, you should leave them there for 20 seconds or so in order to allow ALL the insulin to leave the syringe and enter into the body. If not, you are wasting insulin, as some of it will remain at the point of the needle or remain inside the syringe. If so, it is a waste of insulin and/or a reduced impact, since not all of the intended dosage got into your body.

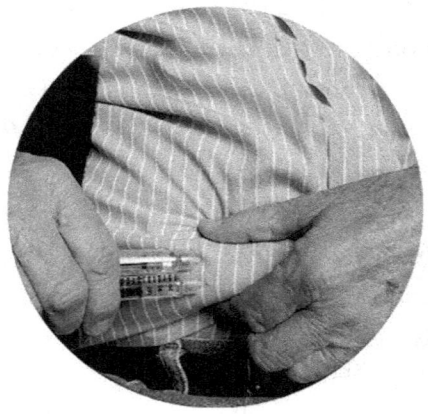

If you can't see clearly, don't have agile hands, and have infections or open wounds, you should not attempt to self-inject, but request that it be done by someone without these limitations

Another technique to save time is to *inject straight through one's clothing* (shirt, T-shirt, blouse, skirt, dress, etc.). This strategy may seem strange and unsafe to many persons. Nevertheless, some diabetics, such as myself, have practiced this technique hundreds and hundreds of times with no negative effects. Of course, the clothing must not be soiled, sweaty or contaminated with other pollutants, as I've described above.

Injecting in the morning before dressing will negate the need to inject through one's clothing; but after dressing and then needing to inject before or after lunch or the evening meal, injecting through the clothes avoids the need to remove the necessary clothing to reach the bare skin. To save time and the repetitive procedure of removing my clothing, I personally have found it much more convenient to simply inject through my garments. But I hasten to declare that I only do it when I am sure my clothing is not contaminated. Some simple experimentation will indicate if this is a process satisfactory for you.

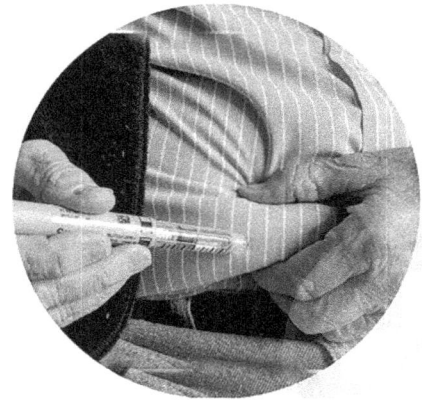

Conclusion

- Type 2 diabetes is a very debilitating disease, which can lead to blindness, heart failure, kidney failure, neuropathy, and impotence; and if not brought under control, some of these can lead to death.
- Fortunately, from official studies, and from actual known cases, it has been clearly demonstrated the disease *can* be reversed. But it should be understood that reversal essentially means that the disease, once brought under control, must be continually controlled, that is, going back to the wrong eating habits, because if not—the disease will return.
- It can't be denied that reversing the disease is a mighty struggle, since eating behaviors are the strongest habits of the human being. But when one has the support of family members, the church pastor, one's doctor, prayer, and God, the habits can be broken. In fact, once the right food and exercise are begun, the blood sugar count will soon get back to normal, and that will bring great delight to the achiever; but more importantly, longer life. It is

possible, despite claims to the contrary, that lancets and pen needles can be used over and over—some have used them more than 100 times—without any adverse results. Since these instruments have very high costs, the savings can become enormous.

- Finding the right body site for pricking and injecting is important, because minimizing pain makes the ordeals much less unobjectionable.

WHIPPING DIABETES

In this section I will address several issues. Each one is important for those who are daily injecting insulin into their body or taking Metformin (or another brand type of the pill)—and struggling with the disease, longing to get it under control. This booklet will help you toward that end.

I will be succinct, that is, keep it short but to the point, and also make it clear, especially for those who may have a short attention span or not able to read lengthy articles due to an eye problem or other negative situations. However, I should point out, that when it comes to one's health, you should not easily abandon material that will definitely improve your well being, so I recommend that you calmly take your time to read this important information, even if it seems a little long to you.

The Danger of Overdosing

One of the dangers of injecting insulin into your body is the possibility of over injecting. How can this occur? As an example, let's say you are used to injecting five units of Lantus and four units of Humalog (or other brand names of both kinds) in the morning, and maybe three units of Humalog at lunch, and three units again at supper, and several units at bedtime; or you may, as I used to do, skip injecting at lunch and supper, and only inject again before bedtime. At bedtime I usually injected five units of Lantus and around three units of Humalog. (The number of units will vary from one person to another.)

However, I actually sometimes varied the amount I injected at bedtime. Why? Because it depended on how much exercise I got during the day, especially in the afternoon. I had discovered from much experience that if I exercised or worked laboriously during the day, especially in the PM for only two to three hours, I had to take a smaller dose of Humalog, or none at all, when I retired for the night.

If not, I would have an enormous plunge in blood sugar count during the night, usually around 2:00 or 3:00 a.m. For some reason or other hardy exercise reduces the body's call for insulin. Let me give you an example. Let's say you have a sedentary job, but one day after work you labored hard in the afternoon doing some type of exercise, either inside on a treadmill or the like, or outside in some type of physical labor in your yard or in some other type of manual exercise. At supper time you ate a piece of pie or other sweet more than you should have of what diabetics should eat.

A couple hours later, just before you go to bed, you take your BSC and come up with a count of 140 or 160, or a bit higher. At this level, you would normally take, for example, three units of Humalog and five units of Lantus (or whatever you are accustomed to be taking).

What I found out was that this is a no no. If you have exercised strenuously that day, and at suppertime ate a bad meal, you must not take any Humalog and maybe no Lantus. More than once, speaking of my personal experience, after working hard in my yard, I failed to eliminate a Humalog injection or by error or through forgetfulness, took the usual dosage, and suffered severely for it.

But I should point out, that if you have got lots of physical exercise that day and your BSC at bedtime is really high, like 175 or above 200, you might take a very small dose of Humalog; but you should probably experiment in order to learn your limits in these situations.

So what happened when I overdosed? I woke up sweating profusely, shaking, feeling weak and very strange, and was aware I had an insulin problem. I immediately took my BSC, and guess what? It was usually way under 80 or 90 and sometimes under 50, and occasionally as low as 43. Scary?

You bet! So what did I do? I always kept beside my bed at least two small boxes of California Raisins and immediately started eating them, both boxes, and in about ten minutes or less, my blood sugar count was high enough to return me to normal. Sometimes I went to the refrigerator and took some cold fruit juice (which usually has some sugar in it) and drank about a glass of it.

I hear you asking "Isn't such a low BSC dangerous? Won't you pass out at that low level?" I can honestly say that I never felt like I would pass out and had never gotten dizzy or felt like fainting. I had probably overdosed about 10 times since I was diagnosed with the disease in November of 2009. In fact, my doctor once told me that a low BSC will not make you faint. I haven't been able to find anything on the Internet that says you will, but it could be that a person with very poor health might. What is my counsel?

Do all you can to avoid such an experience. I might add, if your BSC would go to 20 or lower, it might make you pass out. And be assured, that if this happened to you numerous times, it could damage one of your vital organs, and worse, if no one was there to help you regain consciousness and bring up your BSC, you might die right on the spot.

This leads me to an important recommendation: Always keep several small boxes of raisins by your bed, in your car, and at your work site. And if you travel by plane, be sure to take some with you. They are the quickest and simplest method of bringing up your BSC fast. This is important, because you never know when for some unexplained reason (usually too many sweets) you'll have a drastic drop in your BSC.

By the way, I always kept a Lantus and Humalog pen in the car, and I did the same at my office when I was still

working. I suggest you do the same. It is recommended by the manufacturers of these pens that they always be kept in a cool place; but the ones I kept in our restroom and in the car never failed to be potent.

Relating to Non-Diabetic Meals

One of the challenges conscientious diabetics face is how to relate to food that isn't good for their disease. I faced this many times and admit it isn't always easy to resolve. Let's start with your own home. If you are a child—12 or under—with diabetes, your parents are most sure to do everything they can to give you the best diabetes-favored food. In this case, it's not a problem, although some parents are very negligent, which behavior results in serious health problems for their child.

If you are a teenager, say 15 and above, you are starting to get on your own about the type of food you choose to eat. I am the first one to admit that choosing the right food is a tremendous challenge, especially if you have been raised on junk food, such as sodas and other sweet drinks and lots of carbohydrates and oily foods. To break away from these inappropriate foods for a diabetic is extremely difficult, especially if you have been raised in a family that doesn't have high standards of living; meaning punctuality, organization, cleanliness, and lots of good family discipline.

The problem in this setting is there's no one to work seriously with you to help you eat right and get enough exercise. Primarily, it will be up to your mother to set the right foods on the table and help you carry out these diabetic requirements. But remember, probably the reason you got type 2 diabetes as a teenager is because you were raised in a family that didn't have these high standards. You ate what you wanted with no supervision or discipline, or your parent(s) provided too many wrong things at mealtime.

Or it could be you were raised in a single-parent family with the mother working and leaving you with a babysitter at an early age, and later in your teens you frequently prepared your own meals with the tastiest but wrong foods, and on top of this were influenced by your friends who had a diet contrary to what diabetics should eat.

Another scenario is when your spouse doesn't give a rip about your problem and simply cooks what she (or he) likes, regardless of how it may affect you. She may even contend that the diet you need is not good for the children, and thus place them first. But what she doesn't understand is that **the diabetic diet is perfect for the children, too**. This is a tough one. It can get very sticky, and there's no easy solution. In situations like these, generally there's very little love between the two. The spouse who is abusing is actually killing the partner little by little or bringing about serious permanent bodily defects.

Still another situation is you are indeed careful with your diet, whether as a teenager or a single young adult, or a married middle-ager, or as I am, a senior citizen. You keep it under control, but from time to time you visit friends who either have no idea you are a diabetic requiring selected foods or have other guests who would not be happy with a diabetic meal, or the hostess doesn't really care.

What should you do in this case? Simple. You eat what's set before you, but you eat small servings of what's not good for you and larger servings of what's OK. Why this approach? You don't want to offend your hostess, especially if she and her family are respected friends. What you can do to offset the high count of sugar caused by what you've eaten is to take a shot of insulin in privacy after eating.

Now I hear you say: "How can I do that?" What I personally did to play it safe was to carry my Humalog pen with me when I anticipated such a scene. If you have it in your car, you put it in your pocket when you get out, or put it someplace where it won't be seen. A woman can carry it in her purse. After the meal, I used the restroom or some other secluded place either inside or outside to take my shot. If I accidentally left the pen in the car, I went to the car and took the shot there. From experience you can make a safe estimate of the amount of units you should take. From my experience, I've found it to be the best solution.

How You Get Diabetes

In section 3, I gave you some general ideas about how to overcome the disease. However, I didn't go into a lot of detail because it would have made the reading too long for most people, but there were many good points to consider.

As you may well know, there are lots of books out there for sale on-line about how a person gets the disease, but most of them are long and rather boring. I know, because I've read a number of them. One of them had 75 pages, was not well written, and frankly, was rather dull (but it did have useful info). In this short explanation, I think you will be glad to know how you probably got it. So, stay by and make some good discoveries.

You may recall what I said when I discovered I had diabetes. I told about it in my personal account, My Story. When the nurse came into my hospital room with a needle in her hand and told me she was going to inject me for diabetes, I yelled, "No, that's not for me. I don't need that!" You bet, I was just plain scared.

The next thing I wanted to know, when the reality hit me, was how in the world I got the disease. After some time my doctor came in, sat down by the bed, and did some questioning and explaining. And this is what I want to share with you here.

- **First**, she gave a review of what diabetes is; and I'll share that with you here. I told quite a bit about it in the section My Song. What my doctor said was, that if you have diabetes, it means the sugar you take into your body (through carbohydrates, which turn into glucose—sugar; plus sweet drinks, sweet food such as ice-cream, cookies, cakes, pie, sweet rolls, brownies, etc.) can't get into your cells, which you need for energy, and therefore stays in your

blood stream and causes your BSC to stay too high. This is called hyperglycemia. Such a situation usually causes frequent urination, lots of thirst, and abnormal tiredness; and if not cured, will turn into diabetes and cause eye, heart, kidney, feet, and incontinence problems. The reason your cells get blocked is because you have been eating too much fatty foods. Hence, the challenge for diabetics is to get their cells unblocked so the sugar needed for energy and normal health can enter into the body. By the way, I should also mention hypoglycemia, which means your blood sugar count is too low, usually under 90; but most diabetics don't feel a negative reaction until it gets down into the low 80s or lower. As mentioned above, I've had it down to 43, and that's terrible—sweating, gross tiredness, and shaking. I hope that never happens to you.
- **Second**, she explained that diabetes doesn't come on a person suddenly. It usually takes months or years. In my case, it took years, at least 10, but probably more like 30. Since I am now 80, this means it likely started when I was between 45 and 50. When I was 45 years old, I was overweight. I now weigh 140, but then I was nearly 200 pounds. I had that weight till I was in my early 70s.
- **Third**, she reminded me that it's important to understand that weight alone will not cause diabetes. When I was a boy back in the 1940s and 1950s, I had some overweight friends, but none of them had the disease. In fact, diabetes was hardly ever heard of back then. So, you ask, "How is overweight related to diabetes?"

My answer is that it's not complicated. When you're eating too much of the wrong things, like carbohydrates (sugar) and oily foods (fat) and drinking lots of sodas (more sugar) AND you are overweight, the combination is tremendously problematical and almost always leads to diabetes. The more weight you have, the more insulin you need, but, as I mentioned above, when the cells are blocked from consuming too much fat and thus denying the entrance of insulin into the body cells, the insulin stays in the blood stream and affects several of your internal organs, as I've already mentioned—heart, kidneys, sexual organs, eyes, and even your feet. I repeat this because of how important it is to remember it. These are the things my doctor shared with me and that I was so glad to learn about.

Continuing with the question of overweight, I hear you asking "Why then didn't overweight people get diabetes 50 and 60 years ago? The reason? The food people ate back then was very different than what it is now. And the lifestyles were also different then.

Yes, it's true. Don't go away, and I'll explain. When I was a boy and a teenager, the normal meal for almost all Americans consisted of a wide range of vegetables—green beans, cooked dry beans, carrots, chard, spinach (and other greens), cauliflower, broccoli, lettuce (usually in salads), cabbage, beets, zucchini, white potatoes and sweet potatoes, squash, and some pasta. There was a range of meat also, but mostly pork, chicken, beef and fish. But back then, the meat was different than it is now. Today cattle and other meat animals are fed questionable additions that some experts insist are detrimental to their meat/flesh.

Another important point involves canned foods. At that time there was not the huge array of pre-prepared foods as there are now, and those that were in existence then didn't have as much sugar in them as they currently do. What did people drink back then? Mostly dairy milk and some sodas; Coca Cola, Root Beer, and a few others were popular, but young and older people were usually not addicted to them as so many millions are today.

Additionally, almost all people were getting lots of physical exercise. Since more than 50% of Americans were living in the country, they were busy with farm chores and other daily physical tasks. And those few who were overweight were eating a diabetes-friendly diet.

Even those in the cities were more active than they are now; since not everybody had a car; consequently there was more walking. And another important point is that television and iPhones were not nearly as prominent in homes then as now.

Many people I grew up with didn't have a TV or iPhones; and there weren't as many programs then to glue people to the screen. So, what did they do? They were outside doing various types of work, playing with friends and visiting neighbors. Very few mothers were working then. That didn't start until the mid-seventies. Those non-working mothers were playing with their children, going to the local park, and many were fostering a family garden with the children helping weed, till, and harvest it. I did that with my parents and siblings. Now that lifestyle has all gone with the wind.

Today, with mothers working, the children often fix their own food, food that's diabetes unfriendly. And those children are fixed to the TV and iPhone and eating between meals and consuming all the sweet stuff they can find; and have practically no physical exercise. Millions of teenagers, and even younger kids, are glued to their cell phone. This style is carried into young adulthood and to middle age and beyond. Catching diabetes is just a matter of time. Sadly, many of them are now developing it even as children.

Many who are reading this know what I'm talking about, and, indeed, can trace their diabetes to these roots. You see, the diabetes lifestyle is very complicated. I hate to tell you this, but it's important to know the truth; otherwise it becomes easier to stay in the trap. In the end, a clear understanding of the pitfalls actually makes it easier to beat it.

By the way, let me share a couple of other important things about diabetes problems. It's winter time and you are restricted to indoor life. You were accustomed to getting some outdoor exercise in the spring, summer and fall, but now you can't because of the snow and outright cold. And besides, you're not in love with exercising on a treadmill or the like. To tell you the truth, I'm not a treadmill fan, either. But without exercise you'll automatically have a higher BSC than you should have two hours after meals, unless you are rigid in doing some kind of exercise—like pacing back and forth in your living room—and especially following a very good diabetic diet, even in the wintertime.

If you hate indoor exercise and just can't do it—maybe you can't afford that kind of equipment, or even if so, you don't have room for it; then you need to be exceedingly careful of what you eat. Being rigid with your diet will offset the need to exercise so much; but remember, if you're overweight (I'm not talking about five or 10 pounds, but a lot more) it will be even harder for the rigid diet to keep your BSC under control.

Now I'd like to share with you more about overweight. Most overweight people—I say most, because there are some persons who, because of their genetic makeup, have a powerful tendency to gain weight. The least bit of fatty-type foods will put on more weight for them than it would for most people without this abnormality. So these persons have to be especially careful.

How do overweight people usually gain too much weight? It's usually—but not always—from drinking too many soft drinks per day. Let me give you some data on the amount of sugar contained in sodas and fruit-flavored drinks. As you can see, soft drinks have tons of sugar and tons of calories. Would you pour 15 or even 9 teaspoons of sugar onto a plate and scoop it into your mouth?

12 oz Bottle/Can	
7 Up	9 teaspoons.
Lemon Lime	9½ teaspoons.
Ginger ale 9	½ teaspoons.
Root Beer	11.5 teaspoons.
Colas	11.5 teaspoons.
Cream Soda	12.3 teaspoons.
Grape and Orange flavored sodas	12 to 13 teaspoons.
20 oz Bottle	
Mountain Dew	15 teaspoons

24 oz Bottle	
Sweet Tea	13 teaspoons
Note:	
A 12 oz. can/bottle of soda contains about 140 calories.	
A 20 oz. can/bottle of soda contains about 240 calories.	
A 28 oz. can/bottle of soda contains about 364 calories.	
A 38 oz. can/bottle of soda contains about 512 calories.	

I doubt it. So now it would be way too sweet, and probably repulsive. Of course, I understand that when it's in a liquid form it's considerably more palatable, but that doesn't negate the fact that you're getting too much fat into your system.

Imagine, if you were to drink five sodas per day—which many diabetics, pre-diabetics, and others for whom it's just a matter of time before they come on board, are doing—you would have an average of at least 50 teaspoons of sugar. That's equivalent to 350 teaspoons per week. Are you going to gain weight? Of course—unless you exercise like crazy every day. (But don't forget that excess sugar has other negative impacts on the body.)

According to a study done by Cambridge University, just cutting out one soft drink per day could reduce the risk of developing diabetes by 25%. Many smoothies and juices aimed at children contain up to seven teaspoons of sugar, or 200 ml (milligrams). As an NHS (National Health Service) guideline says, "Added sugars shouldn't make up more than 10% of people's caloric intake per day—70g (grams) for men and 50g for women; and for children it should be less."

WHAT YOUR DOCTOR SHOULD TELL YOU

Besides soft drinks, many diabetics are eating more than enough carbohydrates at mealtime. We all love macaroni, noodles, spaghetti, fettuccini, tortellini, and other similar pastas. We also all love white rice and white potatoes. In large servings, these foods pour an enormous amount of fat—and glucose—into our cells, and make us gain unnecessary weight.

Before we go on to the next section, which deals with the various ways of getting rid of diabetes, I want to share with you what a good doctor should explain to a patient that has been diagnosed with pre-diabetes. Remember what I said in My Story when referring to my experience in Albania when my doctor diagnosed me with pre-diabetes?

You'll recall that he didn't properly explain what I was facing. Probably many doctors don't carefully explain to their pre-diabetes patients clearly enough what they're facing. If your doctor hasn't told you what it's all about, he is remiss. In my opinion, this is what he should say:

Mr./Mrs. Jones, are you aware of what you're facing? Right now you have pre-diabetes. I'm really sorry to tell you that, but this means that your current lifestyle is fostering the disease. You should know that if you don't make changes in your diet and your weight, you'll soon become a diabetic. Do you know how serious diabetes is? As your physician, I want to be upfront with you. It's my duty to tell you. Diabetes is a dangerous disease that can do serious damage to several of your key organs. It can blind you. It can destroy your kidneys. It can give you a heart attack. It can take away the feeling in your feet and legs. And, for a man, it can cause impotence.

It also means that even by controlling it—not letting it get worse—which it's possible to do, you'll still have to take a pill everyday of your life; or worse, if you're careless in controlling it, you'll probably have to start taking shots several times a day, and along with that, prick your fingers each time you inject in order to get a blood sample for determining how much insulin to inject. For some people this is very unpleasant.

The reason I'm telling you these things upfront is because it's important for you to understand the seriousness of diabetes. I can assure you it's nothing to fool around with. But, on the upside, you should know that it can be controlled by a careful diet and exercise.

And for your encouragement, you need to know that it can even be reversed; but to do it, you would have to be extremely careful of what you eat, and lose weight, and maintain a regular exercise program.

If you're willing, I can put you on a plan that can stop your pre-diabetes from becoming full-blown diabetes. Would you like me to do that?"

This is what your doctor should tell you, and if he hasn't told you what I've described above, then you haven't been properly informed. However, if he did tell you and you ignored it, then the responsibility of the disease would not be his.

How to Get Rid of Diabetes

After reading the previous section, I think you're beginning to see the importance of diet—and exercise—in controlling diabetes. But now I will take you into more details about how to actually get rid of it.

- **A1C.** First I have to tell you about A1C. You may already know what it is; however, in case you don't, I'll share it with you, because it's good to know since it's an important indicator of how you are doing with your diabetes. Don't worry about what the actual letters— A1C—stand for. A1C has to do with a blood test to determine your average BSC during the past two to three months. The test measures the amount of hemoglobin in the blood that has glucose attached to it. If there's too much glucose attached to it, there'll be a high A1C. And you don't want that. If you're having some diabetes-type symptoms and have gone to your doctor for an exam, he/she will probably recommend an A1C test. If you have type 2 diabetes, then it's recommended that you have an A1C test done at least twice a year. This is important because it tells you how you're doing with your diet, your exercise, and your injections or pills.

A normal, non-diabetes A1C level is less than 5.7%. A level of 5.7% to 6.4% indicates Pre-diabetes. A level of 6.5% or higher indicates diabetes. If you get up higher than 7%, you can be in serious trouble. At this point, it's clear you need to make some changes in your lifestyle, so don't take your A1C test lightly.

- **Exercise.** Now let's start with exercise. There are many ways to get some movement in your body. Just walking will help a lot. After I got diabetes, my doctor told me, among other things, to walk 30 minutes after every meal. Of course, walking can be done in many places and in many ways, even on a treadmill, as I've referred to already. Exercise is important, especially for grossly overweight persons.

A standing walk can also work. From experience I've discovered that a ten to fifteen minute hard and fast walk on a treadmill, or even a standing one inside the house, can bring your BSC down 20 points. I challenge you to try it. If you have the conditions to do various types of exercise, you can run, but if you are considerably overweight and not accustomed to exercising, then you need to start out slowly and work up to a faster and faster pace. Pushups can also be effective. So can barbells. In fact, any kind of workout can be effective.

You just have to learn where—according to your conditions—and how much you need to do to bring down your BSC. This goes for either slender or overweight persons.

- **Diet.** Next is what you eat and how much. This is what I recommend: eat just one small serving per meal of anyone of the carbohydrates mentioned. Studies done in 2015 have proven that carbohydrates are the biggest cause of overweight, and thus potentially cause diabetes. Drastically reducing carbohydrates—white potatoes, white rice, white bread, and pastas—to mention them again—will make a huge difference in both weight reduction and diabetes. This cannot be overemphasized.

On the rest of your plate have a salad with lots of dark green leafy-type lettuce; plus a variation of carrots, cauliflower, broccoli, a squash of some kind (butternut and acorn are very tasty), dried beans of some variety, string beans, corn—but a small portion, or corn on the cob—only one—all of these cooked; avocado, bell peppers, or some other green vegetable, and cucumbers. There are others (see my list below).

You can eat meat, but keep it to one small piece. Meat is different now than it was 50—60 years ago. Back then, the meat industry was not feeding the animals with non-traditional food and injecting them with growth stimulants; and they were eating pure types of grass (fresh or dried), such as alfalfa and grains, and other sources that weren't from GMO—or chemical-filled ingredients. So, go easy on meat.

A variety of nuts is okay, too, but not too much of any kind, because they have lots of calories. Eat nuts with every meal. I'll talk about this later. Eat lots of fiber. Here's a list of high fiber foods that won't spike your blood sugar:

- **Brown or wild rice, riced cauliflower.**
- **Sweet potatoes, yams, cauliflower mash.**
- **Whole wheat pasta, spaghetti, squash.**
- **Whole wheat or whole grain bread.**
- **High fiber, low sugar cereal.**
- **Steel cut or rolled oats.**
- **Low sugar bran flakes.**
- **Peas or leafy greens.**

For most people, breakfast is when the largest amounts of oily foods are ingested. One of the most common diets for this meal consists of fried potatoes, fried eggs, and fried meat of some kind. I am the first one to admit that fried foods are very delicious, but for the diabetic, they are a big no no; though I must admit that a little now and then—maybe twice a week, but very little and only one moderate serving—is okay.

It's far better to eat a dry or cooked cereal, but only non-sweetened dry cereals and not grits, which United States Southerners love, though perhaps once in a while is okay. I love to eat Raisin Bran, but one must be careful, because this cereal is loaded with raisins. Remember that just one small box of California Raisins is extremely sweet.

Toast at breakfast is fine also, but just one slice from a real whole wheat or multi-grain bread. If you've read the labels of so-called WWB (whole wheat bread), you'll know that most of the bakers fudge, because usually most so called WWB is only 25% or less. A true WWB will be 90% or more and will usually contain several other grains. More than one slice of even a 7-grain legitimate WWB will drive your BSC up some. Avoid using dairy butter and lots of jam or jelly or honey on your bread—all have lots of sugar and fat. In place of dairy butter, use margarines with a low-calorie count.

Nothing sweet to drink—only water or dairy milk, or better, oat milk, almond milk or soy milk. Remember, dairy products are filled with fat. Your biggest challenge will be in eliminating a sweet drink. I know, because I've been through it, but I found that when I stopped sweet drinks (not only at mealtimes), my BSC was much more controllable. Be careful about loading on mayonnaise and dressings on your salads. Many dressings have lots of sugar.

Be careful with snacks. Personally, I never, never eat between meals. Snacking between meals is dangerous. Why? Because snacking almost always implies eating something sweet. Who's going to snack on fresh carrots? Or on cabbage? Or on a cooked potato? And who's going to drink a glass of milk or soymilk, for example, between meals? Snackers almost always snack on sweets. Even a mid-size snack will drive your BSC up 40—50 points. Best not to snack at all. I can guarantee you'll feel better if you don't.

Another habit to watch out for is grazing. What do I mean by this? It's when after you finish your meal you get up and hunt around for various tidbits. I have to confess, I've had this habit, but I didn't look just for sweets, I looked for chips, nuts, sometimes peanut butter (a spoonful), maybe some raisins and other goodies. This bad habit can add unwanted fat that leads to more weight and, worse, a boost upward of your BSC.

Which reminds me, are you suffering from indigestion? Acid reflux? If so, it could be because you're drinking too much with your meals. A lot of liquid dilutes the natural digestive juices in your stomach and thus prevents them—the digestive juices—from breaking down the food; and when this happens, the undigested food turns sour. It has been proven by scientific studies. Most people are not aware of this. If you have acid reflux and are on a medication for the problem, I challenge you to stop drinking with your meals, as well as stop snacking for one week, and see what happens. It may not cure everybody, but I can assure you that it's worth a try.

The 10 best diabetes-friendly foods

1. **Leafy greens**—collard, kale, spinach, chard, mustard, watercress, celery; and in lettuces romaine, green leaf and butterhead (dark-leafed greens are more nutritious).
2. **Green vegetables**—green beans, peppers, cauliflower, broccoli, cucumbers, Brussel sprouts, zucchini, okra, asparagus, artichoke.
3. **Regular vegetables**—tomato, white potato, sweet potato, onion, carrot, turnip, radish, squash, garlic, eggplant.
4. **Beans**—soy, black, pinto, navy, lima, lentil, kidney, chick peas, split peas. Note: Beans are very high in fiber, which is excellent for controlling BSC.
5. **Grains**—whole wheat, buckwheat, quinoa, rye, barley,

millet, spelt, corn, brown rice (all should be non de-germinated/non-processed).
6. **Seeds**—sunflower, soybean, chia, flax, sesame, pumpkin.
7. **Nuts**—almond, walnut, Brazil, hazel, pistachio, peanut, cashew, pecan, macadamia.
8. **Drinks**—soy, oat, almond, dairy (but in small amounts).
9. **Juices**—100% natural is the best kind. There is a large spectrum of these juices with no sugar added. Nevertheless, even one glass of these has a tendency to drive up your BSC.
10. **Meats**—chicken, lamb, beef, all in small servings. Pork is dangerous, since, if not properly cooked, can have trichinella spiralis, which can cause trichinosis, a disease, though controllable, is very difficult to cure, and can kill.

Regarding specific recipes, I recommend you go on line where you can find hundreds of them. **But be careful, there are some touters of how to control diabetes who are confused about what's good and not good to eat.** Some of the recipes are loaded with trimmings that contain too much fat or sweets.

Really? Is it possible? You bet. I'm not talking about 65—70 years old. Anybody can live longer than that. The fact is, you can live a long, long time if you eat right and live right. Of course, there are exceptions, like the minority who are born with certain genetic ailments that the best medical science can't turn around. (Even so, modern medicine can usually help extend their life some and help them live less painfully.)

I'm talking about those persons who have no special birth problems, who have all the normal health advantages. These are the ones who usually get into trouble. Somewhere along the line, usually in their youth, they form habits that ultimately bring about an early death. What are these behaviors? There are at least ten major habits:

1. **Smoking** (Is a deadly habit).
2. **Drinking.** (Can also lead to death).
3. **Drugs.** (Leads to a terrible lifestyle, and can also lead to death).
4. **Overeating.** (Leads to overweight, potentially to diabetes and other diseases).
5. **Awful diet.** (Too much carbohydrates, sugar and oil)
6. **Inconsistent eating.** (Eating between meals and irregular meals).
7. **Dissatisfaction with life.** (Lack of joy and peace).
8. **Laziness.** (Hates work).
9. **Sedentary life style** (Being a couch potato).
10. **Immorality.** (Dishonesty, unfairness, injustice, adultery, etc.).

These are the ten major problems that usually bring about an early death, especially if two or more of these are combined.

The Truth about the Proper Cure for Diabetes

In today's medical world there are not only the well-known pharmacies which produce diabetes control medicines; but also private organizations and individuals who claim non-dietary solutions for curing diabetes. These latter ones can be found on Facebook, in email, and other internet platforms. In most cases, these are scams or non-proven solutions. Though there may be a few isolated cases of curation related to a person's genetic makeup, decades of experience has proven undisputedly that the only true cure is a change of diet from highly saturated glucose foods and sufficient exercise. Of course, it is the prerogative of each diabetic to attempt these non-traditional recommendations if they desire. Experience has shown, however, that diet and exercise are without question the indisputable solutions.

Lamar Phillips

How to Get Rid of Neuropathy Pain

Neuropathy, technically called Peripheral Neuropathy or Peripheral Neuritis, is the result of Diabetes, which damages the peripheral nervous system, that is, the outer layer of skin circulating the legs, usually below the knees, but it can also affect above the knees—and even the hands, according to a description explained in Google. The symptom is manifested by very uncomfortable pain of the skin and can happen over and over again, sometimes every day for days on end. I have had it, and can thus testify to its extreme unpleasantness.

The pain can occur in spots at any place, such as on your ankles, on your legs between the ankles and the knees, and even above the knees up to the hips. Several can take place at the same time on both legs. How do I know? Because neuropathic pain has happened to me in the various places I've mentioned, except above the knees. This is because my neuropathy is not severe.

How does it feel? Basically, it stings or simply has a burning feeling. When neuropathy attacks you, it's really hard to sleep; and during the daytime, it's very distracting, although if you are extremely concentrating on something, you may not feel it, or if so, very little. Eventually, each spot where it is activating will go away. But it will soon be replaced by another attack someplace else on your legs.

So, can neuropathic pain be gotten rid of? Fortunately, it can. What I have learned is that diet without medical attention, can take care of it. When it started on me, several years after I turned off diabetes, or as they say, reversed it, I found the solution, at least a plan that worked for me.

After I originally licked the disease, I was very careful for several years of what I ate. Nevertheless, the numbness in my legs, primarily in my left foot, but lightly though in my right foot, stayed with me, but the numbness didn't affect me. There was no pain. But then, unfortunately, I started eating a number of sweets which I had been avoiding. As a result, neuropathic pain started in on me. I had started eating lots of ice cream, chocolate bars, sweet drinks, and various candies. Oh, they were soooo sweet! I just loved them.

Then one day, a couple of years after those pains started in on me, my wife and I in one year made a major two-week trip to the other side of the United States from where we lived to visit friends and relatives; and that same year we traveled twice to Mexico for two weeks each time, and then we went to Panama and Costa Rica for one month. On each of these trips we ate practically nothing sweet, and because of this I never had neuropathic pain once. But each time when we came back I started in again with those sweets I had been eating and drinking, and the neuropathic pain spots returned. What was my conclusion? Those sweets were the culprit. Now I hear you asking, why didn't diabetes return to you after eating and drinking so many sweets? I thought you said that diabetes is caused by too much sweets.

Believe it or not, but diabetes never returned. How do I know? Because I took my blood sugar count once a week since that year when I kicked it and it varied only between 98 and 124. You see, I wasn't eating sweets ALL the time or eating other diabetes-causing foods ALL the time anymore. It was the periodically eating of sweets for short periods, like four or five days at a time, that brought on the neuropathic pain. What I want to point out, however, is that the reason why I kept getting those painful spots was from my careless eating and drinking those sweet things.

I can't guarantee my solution will be your solution. I only mention it because it is a plan you may want to try IF you are periodically eating and drinking the things I mention here and are having neuropathic pain as a result of it.

Now I need to also point out that IF you are having these pains while having diabetes, then it will continue until you reverse it. But if you have reversed it and been careful with your diet so the disease will not recur, then started eating and drinking sweets for short periods from time to time like I did, and have neuropathic pain as a result, you should discontinue with those short sweet periods. At least give it

Lamar Phillips

a try and see what happens. It's working for me.

How to Live Longer

Have you heard of the Blue Zones? In a study done by Dan Buettner and told in his book The *Blue Zones*, first published in 2008, he tells about seven areas—called longevity hotspots—in the world where people live unusually long lives. These hotspots have more to do with lifestyle than with climate or geography. The zones include, among others, Okinawa, Japan; Sardinia and Acciaroli, Italy; Icaria, Greece; Skane, Sweden; Nicoya Peninsula, Costa Rica and Loma Linda, California.

The amazing phenomena of these spots are how the people live and the ages they achieve. In Sardinia, Italy, the place where people live the longest in the world, according to his study, an incredible number of men reach the age of 100 years. There were 20 centenarians from 1996 to 2016 in that place. In Acciarili, Italy, one-third of its citizens (about 300) live to 80 years old or more. Icaria, Greece, has the highest percentage of 90-year-olds on the planet. And these Ikarians have about 20 percent lower rates of cancer, 50 percent lower rates of heart disease, and almost no depression and dementia. Loma Linda, California also has a very high age-rate—95 and up is common—and a very low level of disease. It's the same on the Nicoya Peninsula of Costa Rica. (See The Blue Zones in Wikipedia for all this data.)

Regarding Nicoya, I can testify to the reliability of what the book claims about this zone, since my wife and I used to live there. Cancer, dementia, diabetes, and other serious diseases were practically unheard of. And 90 years and up was common.

In the United States, healthier living and medical advances have pushed up the average life to 79 (81 for women and 76 for men). Buettner admits, though, that "a strong gene pool is important," but adds that "anyone can gain an extra 12 years. You don't have to take a supplement to do it, or take up jogging." I disagree somewhat with

Buettner here, as I explain below.

What, then, is the secret? It's all about what you eat and drink. There's no other way to put it. But I would add that there needs to be some exercise, not necessarily heavy, arduous muscle work, but at least a moving of the body enough so that the muscles don't get squishy. But remember, if you're overweight, you need to get rid of it, because overweight—as I mentioned earlier—is a contributor to diabetes. And exercise helps.

"These folks [referring to the blue-zone people] eat a high-carb diet." He's talking here about non-refined carbohydrates—bear this in mind. "About 65% of their diet is whole grains, beans and starchy fibers. No matter where you go, the choice of snack is nuts." So, did you get that? If you snack, eat nuts. "People who eat nuts live two to three years longer than non-nut eaters." But don't forget, they have lots of fat, so go easy on them.

What, then, is the secret? It's all about what you eat and drink. There's no other way to put it. But I would add that there needs to be some exercise, not necessarily always heavy, arduous muscle work, but at least a moving of the body enough so that the muscles don't get squishy. But remember, if you're overweight, you need to get rid of it, because overweight—as I mentioned earlier—is a contributor to diabetes. And exercise helps.

Buettner says further that the best ideal diet he found in the blue zones, particularly Nicoya, Costa Rica, was a combination of corn, beans, and squash, because they provide all the proteins necessary for life. And in Okinawa, Hawaii, Buettner says, "Sweet potatoes—high in carotene—fueled centenarians for nearly half of their lives."

Buettner continues regarding drinks—just plain water and herbal green teas improve longevity. According to Buettner's survey, the average American eats about 1,100 meals per year. Just imagine, if a person eats a consistent diet of carbohydrates, oily foods and sweet drinks, how fast unnecessary weight can be put on!

Buettner ends an interview he had with National Geographic by saying that if a person follows the diet of the blue zones people, they can eat what they want two days of the week. He may be right, but the problem with this, as I see it, is the temptation of reverting to the old diet that can easily lead to going back to it permanently. I recommend you don't do it. But if it's a tremendous struggle to you, maybe one day a week is okay.

In another study of eight years, one done by a professor at Loma Linda University, an institution owned and operated by the Seventh-day Adventist Church, begun in 1958 on 50,000 Adventist members, showed that life expectancy at age 35 for Adventist women was three years longer (80 years) than for non-SDA women in California, and that life expectancy at age 35 for Adventist men was six years longer (77 years) than for non-SDA men in California.

It also showed that Adventists had far less cancer of all kinds, less diabetes, and less traffic accidents. Why? Because a large segment of Adventists, who number worldwide more than 25 million today, are vegetarians; and some are vegans. Neither do Adventists smoke nor drink coffee or alcoholic beverages. They are also very easy on drinking non-herbal teas and sodas. And they are heavy on vegetables, and do lots of exercising. In other words, very, very few are couch potatoes.

In 1973, Loma Linda University began on its own a 15-year study comprising 100,000 Adventist members. The results of this study brought out the same results—that the vegetarian diet definitely reduces disease and extends life. For example, those on a high fat/meat diet had a risk of dying almost four times greater than those not on such a diet. Eating lots of fruits and vegetables decreases the risk of cancers of the pancreas, colon, lung, kidney, and stomach.

Furthermore, the study revealed the following:

- Eating nuts at least five times a week gives an almost 50 percent reduction in the risk of coronary heart disease.
- Eating fruit three or more times a week reduces the risk

of lung cancer by two thirds.
- And eating beans, lentils, peas, raisins, dates, or dried fruits at least three times a week substantially reduces the risk of pancreatic cancer.
- Eating flesh foods more than once a week was related to doubling the risk of bladder cancer.
- Men who ate dried fruits three or more times a week decreased their risk of prostate cancer by 40 percent.
- And those who ate whole wheat bread, as opposed to white bread, enjoyed a 40 percent decrease in the risk of a heart attack.

So far you've read some very important things regarding how to overcome diabetes, plus how to live a healthier lifestyle. What you need to do now is make a decision, not merely forget about what you've just read and then say to yourself, "Someday soon I'll get going on this." No, you need to make a plan immediately—a decision to change your lifestyle. What I've shared here is vital for turning your downhill lifestyle onto a much better road.

It won't be easy. But remember, with the help of family, friends, your pastor, God, and lots of prayer, it CAN be done.

MY STORY, CONTINUED

Remembering

In My Story, related at the beginning of this booklet, I told how I got diabetes, how it was discovered, and my reaction to it. I can certainly testify that it was not a pleasant experience. And I know that I share the trauma of such a discovery with millions of other diabetics around the world. Let's face it, diabetes is a very unpleasant disease. But, as we all know, it's brought upon us by our own exceeding carelessness. We can't deny it. Our suffering can't be blamed on anybody else but ourselves.

But I hear you say, "Wait a minute, for me it was done in ignorance. I didn't know what I was doing—that I was eating and drinking the wrong foods. I was only eating what I liked and what was set before me."

To a certain extent you are right. We all eat what we learned from our parents' table. To a large extent, our appetites are formed by what we eat when we are children. This means that to some degree it's what our parents set before us that lays the stage for diabetes. Still, it can be argued that as we become adults we have the freedom of choice, and especially in today's world where there is so much health information available from so many sources, we don't have a lot of excuse for getting into the diabetes mess. Nevertheless, I am not highly critical of diabetics on this basis.

But I have to be honest with you: once you have the disease and clearly know what the solution is, and you refuse to take the necessary steps to bring it under control or reverse it, you are the guilty one. In fact, you are digging your own grave; and, in this situation, *usually* it's nobody's fault but yours. In fact, I definitely blame myself for the diabetes I contracted.

Notice that I said, "Usually." There are some exceptions. For example: your spouse refuses to cooperate in preparing the preferred diabetes-safe foods. Or your financial situation doesn't allow you to purchase the diabetes-friendly foods you need. Or it could be that your physician hasn't given you careful enough instructions of what to eat or not to eat. And it might be you are in a situation that makes it very difficult to daily exercise sufficiently—you are living in a small, uptown apartment building where exercising is a great annoyance to your family or your neighbors. In these cases I am sympathetic with you. It's a tragedy!

For those who have all the right conditions but don't take advantage of them, it's harder to be sympathetic. I know. I've been through it all. Let's be truthful with one another: Controlling one's diet is perhaps the most difficult challenge in the world. Our established eating habits are like a vice clamped on our taste buds. We love to eat what we were brought up eating. Yes, we may make a few changes here and there—add something new or drop a few things; but our overall diet is stable, unchanging. And it pulls at our very guts to make any changes. So, what can be done to change when it's destroying your body? My answer is more of My Story, My Song. I hope it can become your story and your song, too.

Remember, I was diagnosed with type 2 when I was 71 years old. I felt like all hell was falling on me. In my mind, it was the most dreaded disease a person could ever get besides cancer. Pricks and injections, pricks and injections, over and over, never ending until death could take it all away or overcoming it with a strong willpower.

At any rate, with no choice—I thought—I started pricking and injecting, sticking my tummy over and over again, day after day, month after month, year after year. Thousands of times! But, hallelujah, I had some positive things going for me. One was a wonderful, understanding wife who immediately modified our diet to suit my needs. Even though we were already vegetarians, we had still been eating white bread, lots of white rice and white potatoes, and other things that produced too much fat in my body. On oils, we were quite careful. This all took place when we were living in Albania.

About a year later (2010) we retired and returned to the United States and settled down in Eastern Tennessee, on a property with a large front and back yard. During the next four years I worked intensively in our yard, planting flowers, manicuring the lawn, and tending to a vegetable garden. The intensive, daily exercise helped me keep it under control, but not to reverse it.

Some two years later we decided to become vegans. That helped a lot. What is a vegan? A vegan doesn't eat dairy products—milk, cheese, butter, buttermilk, cottage cheese, eggs, or meat of any kind. These have proven to be unhealthy to a greater or lesser degree, depending on how they are prepared and how much is eaten. But it has been proven that one has better health without them.

MY SONG, FINAL

Now that we were vegans, unfortunately, I still had diabetes, though it was better controlled. I was still, however, taking my daily shots of insulin. When I'd taken about 10,000 insulin shots over five and a half years, I learned about a diabetes reversal seminar to be held not far away, so I began attending it with approximately 30 other diabetics. I can honestly say that I didn't learn a great deal of new information about how to control it because I had already done a lot of personal investigation. For me, the most inspiring factor was the group spirit and the challenge the leaders put out to us. By the end of the seminar I had modified my diet still further, mainly eliminating drinking anything at meals and between, except water; and eliminating all sweets except once in a while, and then in very small amounts. I also lost a little more weight: I went from 153 to 140.

Additionally, and I hope you don't mind me saying so, I did lots of praying, pleading with God to give me the will power to overcome some of my critical bad eating habits. The verse in the Bible that helped me most is the one found in Philippians 4:13: "I can do all things through Christ who strengthens me."

Then presto! I did it! Finally, I didn't need any insulin at all. My daily BSC was always around 90 or so in the mornings and just above 100 at bedtime. I was thrilled. But guess what! Of the 30 or so who attended, I was the only one that reversed it. Don't get me wrong.

Lamar Phillips

I'm not bragging. In fact, I'm almost crying. Why? Because the fact that the other 29 failed indicates how difficult it is to beat the disease, or it demonstrates that most diabetics are not frightened enough or not wishful enough, but sufficiently satisfied with the pill or needle routine, to not take change very seriously. Or it could be that their home situation was extremely difficult to accommodate their situation. And it could be they are not pleading enough with God to help them.

Some of you who are reading this may not be Christians, but whatever the case, you and I know it's a tremendous challenge, and only special aid—whether it be your spouse, your physician, or your closest friend, or God, can help us overcome it. So, if you haven't tried God, why not attempt it? You have nothing to lose. But remember, God doesn't always answer on the first try. He sometimes wants to test your faith. So don't give up. Keep on praying until it works.

So now I hear you saying, "What's your song?" I was hoping you would ask that, because it's something I'm eager to share with you. I hope it's a song you, too, one day soon will sing with me.

MY SONG by Lamar Phillips

Dreamed to be free, oh, free at last!
From a plague that came on me,
And hit me, hit like a blast.
Shot my blood to a BSC,
Out of sight and out of control,
Till my health and my hope,
Were gone from from my soul.

Longed to be free, yes, free at last!
From a plan that'd come to me,
That'd leave me, free at last,
And bring my blood to a BSC
From out of sight to under control
Till health and yes hope
Would be found in my soul.

Then a plan that I did at last,
Took my insulin from tender me.
Hallelujah, the die was cast:
No more gauge for a BSC,
Nor a nickel from my wallet,
Since my health and my hope
Gave them a wallop.

So now my friend, I've finished my task.
A plan, a plan that set me free.
Hallelujah, did it fast.
Did it now, and am filled with glee.
Diabetes under control,
And my health and my hope
Are at peace with my soul.

www.ingramcontent.com/pod-product-compliance
Lightning Source LLC
Chambersburg PA
CBHW030220121125
35326CB00050B/1051